Born in North London in 1₵ ＿₵nⱺgnue was a miracle child, surviving a major heart operation. The success of this operation has been a benchmark of his determination to succeed in life and persevere when the going gets tough. Married with three children, he runs a successful plumbing and heating company, communication being a top priority between himself and his customers. His love of communication has led him into book writing, with a deep understanding of his own personal circumstances. It is time for him to share a new gift, the miracle and understanding of self-improvement as he knows it.

My inspiration for this book has come about by asking the deep profound question which has been asked for millennia: "Who am I? And why are we here?"

This question, in part, must be dedicated to my brother, who sadly passed away. His passing in 2014 has led me to try to understand myself on a deeper level. In the years gone by since his passing, I have fallen on some hard surfaces, the desire to improve myself and live life to my truest and best potential has given me the craving to learn.

I have to also dedicate this book to my wife and my father.

My wife has stuck by me through thick and thin, and has always encouraged more for me, never listening to the excuses and forever pointing me in the right direction. It can honestly be said I owe the woman I married way more than the dedication I can write in this book. I love her with all my heart and will forever be grateful for the love she has given me.

My father has instilled in me the work ethic, the courage to continue when things are tough and the strength to persevere. I owe my dad the greatest thank you for raising me in such a way which helped me become the man I am today.

Steven O'Donoghue

UPGRADE ME

AUSTIN MACAULEY PUBLISHERS™

LONDON • CAMBRIDGE • NEW YORK • SHARJAH

A CIP catalogue record for this title is available from the British Library.

ISBN 9781528999304 (Paperback)
ISBN 9781528999311 (ePub e-book)

www.austinmacauley.com

First Published (2020)
Austin Macauley Publishers Ltd
25 Canada Square
Canary Wharf
London
E14 5LQ

I would like to acknowledge all the experiences and people spoken about in the book which have helped me understand myself on a deeper level; this in turn has helped assist me in the understanding of helping people make real changes in their life.

I am grateful to Austin Macauley for all the hard work and dedication in helping me get this book out from the midst and into the open. Their assistance and belief in this book have helped raise its awareness to the masses and for that I am tremendously thankful.

Introduction

My passion for the everyday person to improve, be better human beings, understanding themselves and their potential has risen from my own depths to create a new me. I have discovered that life as a whole works best when you are in tune with yourself, your thoughts and feelings are united and there is a wholeness and balance which is distinctly your own. Life can seem like an endless circle of problems sometimes; it can often be hard to see the wood from the trees and blaming yourself becomes, well, part of the problem! In this book, I would like to share with you what *Upgrade Me* is all about, how I see life should be for the everyday man and woman who seek improvement and learn to notice their own uniqueness, the blessings you should be recognising in order to feel grateful and learn to be content with life. If things get on top of you on a daily basis, the visions of a better life may be waning into the abyss. If you have a problematic lifestyle and it makes you feel depressed and you wished for something more but it seems impossible, the wish for a magic button you could press and boom it is all how you could imagine it to be, well this could be the book that gives you a new perspective.

No point in looking at things from only one perspective when you have a mind that can view it from many.

Question time, how questions enlighten you!

The possibility of upgrading one's self? A question which entered my mind in the early stages of 2017. I needed to improve, so I embarked on a quest of how to do this! The first thing I first thought was, *I wish I could upgrade*. Can I change in such a way that indeed it would be a form of upgrade? Yes, is the answer, this is entirely possible, and must for growth, a must for self-improvement.

Just like computer software being installed to replace the old, slow and out-of-date (ways of thinking) programme driving your computer (body), its capabilities have become exhausted because it is stagnant. Are we not the same? How do we consider ourselves to be, to have become, who we are? Most people would describe their personalities, which is of course not wrong, this is who they are, but I would suggest that a lot, not all people, are not entirely happy of who they have become, who they are. Just a bit like the computer analogy, we have some suppositions of our own life. We get out what we put in, how many times we have heard that growing up as a child. This is a belief system which some parents try to instil in their children to help them succeed. So, work hard, put the effort in and you will see the results. So, if I was a computer programmer for instance and I've got a certain idea – I will build my programming around this idea, the patterns of the programme, its fundamentals, are already pre-determined because the programme follows a set of strict rules (subconscious beliefs). This programme is given a name, (windows) (your characteristics, happy, moody, positive, negative) and it becomes recognised and it is used further and copied (passed down to our children). Over time this programme becomes exhausted, (overused, repeated behaviour) overused and generally outdated. So, we go out to our local computer store and buy a faster and more efficient model of the old programme. It's as simple as that, well if you're a computer. But let us not forget, we are the ones who design these computers, so what can we design for our own lives. Is it time to upgrade? Design your life for you! You choose your upgrade, you choose everything!

First off, we need to look at ourselves to "buy a programme" for ourselves. A programme for us is nothing more than new knowledge, a new way of thinking, as my science teacher (Mrs Kelly) once told me, knowledge is power. So, by looking at ourselves, we can begin to understand how we have become the person we see. What knowledge do we currently have? Who taught us this knowledge? Ask yourselves these questions and take time to reflect over them.

We need to truly understand ourselves in order to achieve a complete upgrade. By upgrade I mean to become better, to grow, to improve your being! Know thy self. Finding out who we are or what has come of our lives will require some serious honesty! To one's self at least! This brutal honesty will help you to bring into the light the aspects of you that will require "deleting".

Now it's not a bad idea to have an image in your mind's eye of your ideal self – *The Upgrade.* But to truly upgrade we must first get rid of all our outdated programmes that make up our habits, behaviours, moods, lifestyle etc. So, ask yourself firstly, why do I want to upgrade? Be honest with yourself but remember this is not a time to beat yourself up. This is just a reflection of one's self (with honesty). If you look into a mirror, you see an image; now think, if that image was made up of words, what would you be seeing? Don't be harsh, be honest, looking at this way you are telling the truth, which is a good characteristic to have as a part of your new upgrade. So, get the practice in!

A list of words you might see in a reflection should be unique to you, no one else's opinions are necessary here so don't let that be a part of it. If you are fortunate enough to be able to read this book with your own eyes, you have the intelligence to understand and conceive the idea of an upgrade, let me tell you, that is just part of the remarkable mind you have. Rendering old ways of being, old programmes, beliefs, habits and behaviours is entirely possible. However difficult you may think it is.

Bite-Size Me

So, we understand to acquire an upgrade we need to understand who we are currently. By grasping who we are we can fully focus on the aspects of ourselves we want to develop, keep or erase from our being.

For example, you envisage yourself being slim, perhaps with a six pack, (male or female) a fully toned muscular body – this is your "upgrade". Invariably by wanting this type of upgrade, you're unlikely to be slim already. So, you're likely to be overweight, this is obvious. But what is the overweight person in the mirror behaving like on a daily basis, and more importantly, why? You eat irregularly, you eat the wrong types of food – high calorific dense food with little or no nutrients. Where did this person come from; are you confident or are you shy? Are you in a relationship or are you single? Are you overworked, are you stressed, are you even employed? You see all these other factors in your life play a part to who you are – how you've come to be what you see, what is your environment, the job you have, the people you mix with? And of course, these examples are for you to be able to get your brain ticking the right way, but there could be many other different reasons or scenarios. It may stem from your childhood, a tragedy, poverty etc.

Why am I like this; why do I want to change/upgrade? Is this change a natural innate feeling from within? Is there a strong sense of unknowing and a strong desire to understanding yourself and feeling there must be more to your existence than there currently is?

The first key is finding your "why"! So, break yourself down into some bite-size chunks in order to evaluate yourself.

Make a bullet-point list of who you are, this will give you many trails of thought, it will help you see yourself objectively. This exercise can be painful, it can bring up parts of your past you would rather wish to forget – but it will help you to discover your "why". Why am I this way?

When I discovered my "why", I found it a lot easier to make changes in my life and "upgrade". Personal experience, which I will talk about later in the book, gives me the passion to help people to discover themselves and upgrade.

Upgrading is my passion, and I want it to become yours. The word in itself is inspiring and conjures up the feeling of positivity. You only must think about material pleasures of upgrading i.e. your phone, your wardrobe, your TV or indeed your TV package, to know the feeling you get. But for many people they want to upgrade what's around them to feel good, rather than look inside and get down to the nitty gritty to make the changes within themselves.

You must learn the feeling of contentment and understand it. External pleasures can give us a wonderful (short-term) feeling, but to be truly happy from within, contentment is key. Contentment would be the basis, simplistic things bringing you joy, ultimately gratitude for the things in life which are truly important and for which you are probably unaware are in abundance in your life; you just can't see them because they are out of focus, your perspective is focused on other things!

"Upgrade yourself today," almost sounds futuristic, doesn't it? But imagine a human upgrade shop on the high street, what would you go in and ask for if money wasn't an object. Think about that!

Some examples of looking at yourself objectively, in a bite-size me chunk list may look like this:

Remember, the list is designed for you to figure yourself out on a deeper level to help you find "your why", no one else's.

Who-am-I list:

1. I like to drink – why?
2. I like to smoke – why?

3. I like to socialise with a certain group – why?
4. I like to watch sports and drink alcohol – why?
5. I like spirituality – why?
6. I like Jesus – why?
7. I like nice things, materialistic – why?
8. I like money – why?
9. I like thrill-seeking – why?
10. I like my job – why?
11. I like art/drawing – why?
12. I like a certain team – why?
13. I like reading – why?
14. I like the sound of rain – why?

Can you see? How many of these "likes" are internal (contentment) pleasures, and how many of these "likes" are external.

As you can see, I have used the words "I like" at the beginning of each sentence followed by a descriptive word. This is then followed by a "why" question. I believe in saying "I like" first instead of the very powerful "I am" phrase because this is how people base themselves, on their likes! This is what makes them believe who they are. However, just because someone says, "I like to drink," does not mean it isn't an issue in their lives, or that they do not drink too much, or it affects them in certain aspects, impacts them in certain areas of their lives.

Everybody "likes" certain things and some things are a benefit to our lives, however some "likes" have become attachments within us and formed some habitual behaviours which are detrimental to our being, our true selves. Our "likes" are not necessarily "us". And by deconstructing our "likes" and false beliefs we can understand ourselves on a deeper level and make positives changes. In penetrating these specific points and asking "why" I like this or "why" do I like that we can delve that bit deeper into our "likes" and perhaps discover some hidden truths. The subtle way about this is that you can write stuff about yourself that may have formed some negative patterns, habits and behaviours in your life without feeling, or indeed writing, you hate yourself!

Upgrade me is not about hating yourself, it is most definitely about loving yourself, and I mean your actual "self", not your "likes". Even if your likes make you feel uncomfortable because you so desire to change it, you must still have liked it at some stage if only for the most trivial of reasons, it still became a part of your life (likes). Remember this, your "likes", even if attached to negative feelings for you, are **"not you"**.

Be defined by the visions that will shape your future, not by the memories that tainted your past!

Time for Another Phone

Can you imagine holding onto the same phone for five years. Wow, five years in this day and age, your phone will be very dated. Imagine this, your phone would have been dropped and bashed countless times, looking rugged, scratched and battered on the surface. Internally, the phone's storage would be bursting at the seams with data, images, videos, messages, contacts etc. Everything will be screaming at you "upgrade" me! So you say to yourself – right, time for a new phone – what's the latest model that would best suit my requirements? Your life here requires you to change at different stages, don't hang onto things that do not serve you. Having new knowledge and not making the changes necessary is nothing more than cognitive dissonance.

Now, for argument's sake, imagine this: you're 10 years back in time, it's 2007 and you like many different things. Some positive and some negative but fundamentally you were doing okay in life, you were in cruise control. Now it's 2017 and you are, fundamentally, still the same person. No change. Still in cruise control (blindly). For me at least, to coin a phrase of the times, I would say that is #boring. Upgrade me is like constantly refreshing the pages, and the tabs open on your phone. You need to be constantly moving forward and striving for the growth within yourself. Never neglect yourself at the expense of anyone else or anything else. You deserve a better you today, so "upgrade"! Take note in life, make a bite-size-me list and start today, "now"! You are capable of a lot more than cruise control, bad habits, poor behaviour and constantly falling into traps of repetitive shortcomings.

It's on You!

One thing in this life of ours we must always be aware of is our actions. Actions have consequences! I hope the action of reading this book is a very positive one. We have a responsibility in this world to be our best. Nothing, absolutely nothing, will magically give us our best, we must find it deep within ourselves. It is a full-time job, unpaid and sometimes unappreciated. But let me tell you from personal experience, it is the best feeling, working on yourself daily to "upgrade"! Practise saying to yourself each morning, 'I am going to be the best me I can possibly be today.' Saying this sentence will automatically get you thinking positive. Thinking positive will help you think the very best thoughts, feel good, act good and coincidentally be good! You can then start eradicating those "likes" which formed such a big part of your life from a negative standpoint and start "upgrading" to the more authentic you.

Imagine this conversation!

'Hello sir, can I get all these bad habits removed and can I upgrade to these new habits please?'

'Of course certainly, that will be £150 then, step this way.'

Remarkably, I haven't managed to invent such a wonderful way of upgrading one's self just yet, as nice as it sounds. Perhaps one day there will be "upgrade me" shops up and down all our major highstreets in all our major cities. For people who feel fed up with who they are, what they are doing and the path they are currently on, a one stop shop sounds perfect. Focusing on all your upgrade needs and requirements. Primarily focusing on the state of your mind and the attention to thought patterns and behaviours which are causing you struggles, and you wish to change/upgrade. This shop will be the place to go, also with some exclusive spas, treatments, fitness, hairdressing, you name it, it's "upgrade me" time.

Individually all these things exist, they're just not all in the same place and under one banner. 'It's on you' to make the changes required to upgrade your life, there is no easy path, and no one stop shop or easy short cut (as much as I would love for there to be a one stop shop one day).

As I said in the previous chapter it's key that you find your "why" to upgrading. The true answer to you will be astounding. It will be your driving force into making permanent positive changes to your life, the upgrade. A new you will literally come out of it, that's exactly why it's an upgrade. Old ways of being, poor thinking, lack of self-belief will fade away into the abyss.

Completely abandon old ways of thinking today, get new insights and new skills, practise self-discipline and self-mastery and attain great life-changing results, attain your upgrade – "it's on you"!

You don't have to be that shadowy being anymore, and speculate the possibilities of the upgraded version of you, hold those wonderful images clear in your mind and make them real. Knowledge is power to our being, so fill yourself with plenty of it, read, read, read and read some more.

Be aware of the endless possibilities you hold within yourself, and stop letting fear of change be the ruler of your heart and internal guide. If you always say no to an opportunity of change, you are limiting yourself to possibilities of a new reality. By being open minded and gaining control of the fear that strikes up when opportunity comes your way, you can be open to all possibilities that life can offer you.

Poor thinking will always hold you back, and neglecting your mind is like abuse. Neglecting your mind will cause ongoing pain and suffering, then you will repeat the process automatically to affirm your own beliefs/likes, and around and around you go, before you know it, it's 10 years down the line and the proverbial crap is still flying of the fan in the same room, you haven't changed.

It's on you, always has been and always will be. The blame game is a very common excuse as to why you can't make a change. Often the blame lies away from you, doesn't it? It's because of this circumstance or because of that circumstance. You know the pattern. Well I'm afraid to say, circumstances are what occur all around us daily. So, either you effect the circumstances, or you let the circumstances affect you. Poor thinking in an "unfortunate situation" will only perpetuate feelings of negativity. Keep yourself 100% aware of the upgrade (be conscious of your thoughts and the behaviour you are expressing) always to limit the loss of control of your thoughts.

Fear Projections

Your mind has this wonderful ability to keep you safe; an automated system that works in such a way, it will fill your body with adrenaline to prepare you to run or to prepare you to fight. This is called the fight or flight response. This happens within milliseconds of an emergency situation that will help keep you safe; this is designed in such a way that you don't have to logically think about what to do, just like a zebra or a gazelle does not have to think to run from a preying lion. Imagine you could have the opportunity to think about an emergency, what would you call an emergency? Now, would you really want to have to think about it?

The school bully is a great and relatively simple (human) example, it is now his (or her) turn for some new fresh pickings, and you're the target. As the approaching bully is heading your way, you almost instinctively know this encounter is not going to be friendly without a word even being spoken; the energy for which you can detect coming from this person is not positive in the slightest, and you are immediately filled with adrenaline which is based on the fear from those negative energies you detected. The encounter ensues and it is highly likely, the fight or flight response has kicked in. You either fought back in some form with adrenaline-infused blood rushing around your body, or you used all that highly dosed pumped up blood to kick-start your legs like a formula 1 race car and get out of there.

Your conscious mind does not have to account for this automated response and is taken over by the subconscious, which kicks you into gear and off you go, whichever the response may be!

Your mind has the ability to also project fears into your thinking which affects your decisions. This is almost like the override as in the aforementioned, however it is more to do with prediction of future events to keep you safe rather than an emergency situation. Interestingly, you can control this, and it is important you do so. The reason I want to make this a topic is because I believe it is essential you are aware of this attribute you have, and how there are distinctively different types which reside within you and the one you need to be mostly and acutely aware of is the one you can control, with some conscious thought and practice. Learning to control this is not necessarily easy, as some of the fear projections your mind throws your way does genuinely have your safeguarding as its best interest. But I have managed to notice there is a balance that needs to be achieved in order to serve your "upgrade me" status.

Let me give you an example of my own in where fear projections came into play, and admittedly with some help (as this was my own first time being aware of it and overcoming it) everything fell into place and thankfully I was in a better place.

I was looking for work after being made redundant from my job (at a plumbing and heating firm) and I found an advert for a plumber doing site work. The site in itself was not a brand-new tower block being thrown up but rather a full refurbishment job in an old, large Victorian house in Central London. I went for an induction to the site and was asked to do the installation of the main 4" stack waste pipe work. I persevered with this for about a week or so when the foreman of the site approached me and asked me, 'Can you do copper pipe work, boilers and hot water tanks?'

I basically responded with, 'Well, I am qualified to do all that.' He then proceeded to show me the entire plan for the job (never seen architects' plan for a job this size in my life). I went home that night after my shift and was met with some serious fear projections of the mind. What if this happens? What if I can't do it all? What if I make a mistake? What if it all goes wrong and they blame me and sue me?

For the life of me what was I thinking! I am a fully qualified plumbing and heating engineer. I spoke with my then fiancée (now my wife I can happily say) and she said what are you worried about? The conversation went along the lines of all my fears I had projected into the future events of that job. I was struck with fear and could not make a decision (fear projections). The advice which I still remember to this day was, 'don't look at the entire plans of the job, do one bit that you need to do, complete it and move on to the "next".

I took the advice, got control of my fear projections and made the decision to take on the plans for the job (under the advice of, one bit at a time). Six months later, I completed the entire house, everything from top to bottom was all my installation, five floors of plumbing, bathrooms, toilet rooms, kitchen, boiler and plant room, shower rooms, all my work. My confidence went through the roof. Trust in my own ability was untouchable. Following the end of that project, I was put in touch with another plumbing and heating firm from one of the guys on that site, and I worked for that lot for five years. My world was synchronised and working for me. I keep that simple bit of advice now for every job I undertake, not all big ones either, because when things go wrong you need a plan and you can't give into your fear projections and panic; just one bit at a time and perseverance, you'll get there. Simple but very powerful when implemented. Remember the story of the tortoise and that hare?

The moral of my short story on fear projections is, recognise that sometimes your fear projections are just trying to keep you in your comfort zone and not safe, although safety is what it will feel like. And you could be limiting yourself from that "upgraded" version of yourself which is actually lying there ahead of yourself in the future, but it is for you to choose the path. Be conscious of the fear projections your mind plays out in order to keep you in your comfort zone, it limits you. *Upgrade Me* does not allow for limiting beliefs. Keep yourself humble, but always know you are special and can achieve a lot more than you think.

Coming Away from Yourself

You will find, in order to make an upgrade you will need to come away from yourself. By this I mean your "old ways". I refer to them as old ways purely because that is exactly what they will become once you have upgraded yourself. So, as I wrote in the previous chapter, speculate the new versions of yourself – the upgrade. Immerse yourself deep in the thought of that person you visualise as the new you, now you will realise the "old ways" cannot possibly remain on any level in order for that new upgraded version of you to rise up and come forth. The whole point of the upgrade is to become a better you, so this will be different for every person in both the "old ways" and the "upgrade me" version. It will be different for everyone, what you want to upgrade, what old ways you need to abandon in order to attain the upgrade. It's all unique to you!

Slowly start to adjust your behaviour to mirror this new upgraded version of yourself. So, you will need to have a clear image of this upgrade in your mind. Now like before, if that image was to reflect words back to you that was attached to characteristics and behaviours – what would you see? – list them! Now once you have made that list, hold it and keep it close. Make sure you can see it every day, and repeat to yourself each day, how can I be the best me today? Look at your list and work on one point of a characteristic. This is to focus your attention fully and help you master one point at a time on your list. Remember, this is a work in progress not an instant coffee. As it is a work in progress, be aware of your progress also. Take notes of your achievements, for example, if you normally drink a bottle of wine every evening with a takeaway and you felt this was an area you would like to adjust, to upgrade, then list your achievements in this area i.e., no alcohol with a meal for two weeks and home cooked dinners are now five times a week, regularly.

Keep making these achievement's lists to overview your progress. Build up that new sense of self-belief and new-found confidence. "Yes", "yes", "yes", you are upgrading yourself. Each time you overview your list, you are becoming a step closer to your upgrade.

There is no sure-found way to upgrade, because simply everybody is different. But what you must always keep in mind is the analogy of the computer programmes or the mobile phone. With these you know what you have, they then become dated, so you search for the upgrade you so desire. It's that simple to explain. In practice, it's very different of course. But you can do it, you can become that upgrade whatever it shall be in your mind. Build up some trust in yourself. Build up an overpowering belief that you can concur anything that stands in the way of you and your upgrade – even if that is yourself! And if that is yourself, you need to come away from yourself. Because a new version of you is awaiting, it's calling out to you to upgrade, just like your outdated old phone in your pocket. Make a deal with yourself to go with the flow on this, and trust the process of the "upgrade"!

A key factor in any endeavour is your enthusiasm and your positivity, 'You can do anything if you have enthusiasm', Henry Ford. These two attributes are intertwined and woven together, exclusively. Upgrading would not be possible without them. Why? Well in terms of an upgrade, it's an improvement, correct? So therefore, any improvement from whatever place you are coming from on this (personal to you) will lead you to somewhere more positive, hence being positive. Positivity will breed enthusiasm for what you are doing, thereupon paving the way for more positivity to enter your daily life. It will stand to reason that you will need to delve deep within yourself to conjure up that minute amount of positivity you have lying around within, for the cycle of positivity and enthusiasm to grow. It may take some time to find this from within, especially if you are at a particularly low point in life.

But fear not, because you are great! And whatever you think of yourself right now, when you have gotten down to the nitty gritty from taking a close look at yourself you will come to realise, above everything else – you can change you. "Upgrade me"! This is now your anthem to dance to daily. "Upgrade me", "upgrade me", "upgrade me" – you get the idea.

In times of personal growth and change, you may find yourself oscillating back and forth from the new you to the old you. I found this pretty normal in my growth period and change. I would dip my toe in with full assurance that this is where and who I wanted to be, then boom! I would do something that pulled me straight back into my old self (almost like stepping into the past). I now view this as a positive and natural part of the process, it's almost as if there is a thin layer between the new upgraded version of yourself and the old you, and you can oscillate between them. If you find yourself here, if this sounds familiar, then you can only be on the right track. Perseverance is key. Each time you go back it gets more and more painful, as the realisation of the new you is within grasp. As you get closer to the new upgraded version of yourself, you oscillate to the point where you are physically propelled into the new you like an Olympic shot put thrower spinning faster and faster until the heavy ball is released, never to return to that spinning cycle, and the oscillating period is over! No going back! That thin layer between, is now well and truly shut. You are upgraded to a version of yourself that is authentic.

What Right Do You Have to Be Miserable?

Upgrade Me has been written for people to find inspiration within. There is no science (well I suppose everything is some kind of science) here or crazy gimmicks to lead you down a path to which at the end of it is a brand-new upgraded version of yourself. There are many books out there that need to be read as part of your own journey to "upgrade". As I said, knowledge is power, so fill yourself with it. *Upgrade Me* is my concept (way of putting it) to help inspire people to consciously do and be better. The famous Florence Scovel Shinn, an American artist and book illustrator once said, 'You can control any situation if you first learn to control yourself.' Very true indeed.

Take time here to review a situation you know you could have done better in if you only controlled yourself. I have certainly had many of them I wish to forget. *Upgrade Me* is your road map to better thinking, positivity, and a realisation of how special you are. I am not a teacher of these, but if you're not already, I would highly recommend practicing into your daily routine, meditation and mindfulness. Also, seeking out inspirational people who will help you see the ball in the game from a different perspective.

Tetra-amelia syndrome is a rare disorder characterised by the absence of all four of your limbs. There are men and women in this world who have this incredibly debilitating syndrome and yet still refuse to be cowed by the harshness the world can throw at them. Why? Because they still have the power of their minds and use it. Nick Vujicic, an inspirational speaker and author born with this debilitating syndrome is without a doubt an exceptional man who has, by my own words, upgraded himself (his mind set). As I said previously, the upgrade for which you so desire will be different for everybody, but always know this, you have a purpose. Nick Vujicic has focused on the positive rather than the negative which in turn has given him purpose through his work, and recognition throughout the world.

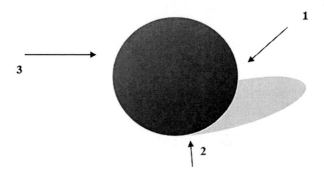

I have drawn a very simple spherical ball shape to illustrate how things are often seen in life when in terms of mindsets. There are three observers of the same ball but only one can see the side that is not lite the most, viewer 3. The ball is always a ball, it just depends on how you view it. It's up to you to move through your obstacles (around the ball to the other side) to get a different perspective of the ball (life) Nick Vujicic would be in the viewer 3 category of people in this world, yet I can assure you he would have had to move from viewer 1 to viewer 3, but he did it. And so can you.

See opportunities – not obstacles, move up, not down, stay in the light not the dark. And never be a realist; this mindset allows you to view things with very limited vision and keeps you stuck in your tracks to stay the same because your too fearful to step out of your comfort zone. In fact, it's easier to move from straight negative to positive as sometimes things are so dark (bad) you have no choice but to make that jump to change (upgrade) and there is only one way to go from there – into the positive – into the light.

My own life experiences would be challenging by anybody's standards. The loss of my mother as a six-year-old boy, the breakdown of my first serious relationship from which my son was born, the death of my brother when I was 27 years old, himself only 34. These are just a few examples of some of the curve balls life threw straight at me and my family. But it has been through some tough, very close analysis of myself that I have swung myself through the obstacles and challenges facing me; that I have been able to "upgrade me".

To get through to making a real change, I have had to get rid of some very poor habitual behaviours of my own. My wife would hate it when I would tell her I was coming home after work on a Friday only for me not to turn up until early Saturday morning, or sometimes afternoon. I would tell myself all the excuses under the sun, the deaths in my family, the area I was brought up in and the like, to reaffirm to myself the lies I was truly telling myself. But all the while I was suppressing the tiny little voice within telling me to change. 'You don't like doing this, this is not you, change'.

Yet speaking to many people including psychologists, I could not grasp any real meaningful change on a consistent level to help myself and my relationship. I was looking outside of myself for change, instead of the most important place, within. It took time to analyse myself, it was a skill I had to practise daily almost, to find a breakthrough for me to make a change – to upgrade.

So what reason is there for you to continue to be miserable? Because challenges, obstacles and life curve balls will come whether you want them to or not. So why not take back some control and some power and "choose to upgrade".

Sometimes it can be hard to see that your life requires an upgrade, and remember, this is not materialistic. But it's never hard to feel it needs an upgrade. Let's be honest, how many of us bury our emotions and cover the feelings of anguish, pain, suffering and guilt to just keep face in all that we've ever known; from people to places, we stay in the comfort zone! Ironic we call it our comfort zone, because it actually causes us more long-term pain and suffering than the actual pain process of change does. Why would you deny yourself your best self? Because that's what you would be doing for a lifetime if you never choose to upgrade! My whole life has changed since I choose to ask myself that simple question (The possibility of upgrading one's self?)

For me, there was a "feeling" I wasn't quite in the zone from which my guise was outwardly expressing to all that was around me! I couldn't see the wood from the trees, but I most certainly feel all wasn't as it should be. I suppose you could call it an awakening, gentle nudges to say, 'hey, wake up, what are you doing?'

So, from that one simple question, taken seriously of course, has led me to many questions and self-discovery. Ultimately with the goal of upgrading, sometimes you don't need to know the whole path, just start where you're at and let go. Trying to create all the scenarios in your head like a road map of: what if this happens, I'll do this and what if that happens, I'll do that. This is a killer, you will put so many excuses and obstacles on that path yourself through projection of your own fears, you will never embrace the journey of change and upgrading. You must trust in a process that's greater than yourself and do the minute things on a daily basis which make you "feel" like you're in accordance with your upgrade. Take what you value in life and blow it up so big everyone can see it. I am living in pure gratitude for life now, I love life, not just my life, but the whole experience. I am humble to my blessings and grateful for everything that I am, everything I have been, everything I am yet to become; gratefulness for all that is and all that will be.

G:- greatness can be achieved by
R:- relinquishing the
A:- access of our external senses and
T:- through the use of the
I:- internal
T:- thought process (meditation) you can
U:-unify the

D:- dimensions from within
E:- equally, heart and mind become one.
Wholeness is generated.

My life is in accordance and balance, and for me, gratitude has been a significant tool which I have embraced and learnt to use, like acquiring a skill. I have honed in on it on a daily basis that it is now a make up in the fabric of my DNA. It's now an automated programme which brings amazing life coincidences and synchronicities.

Michael Jackson's song, *The Man in the Mirror*, this is a perfect example of changing the world, but it starts with you. Your upgrade. I can't physically help all the people in this world who are suffering, but if we can significantly change ourselves, then we can teach our children different. And to be more like the change which they see in us, and with a little luck and perseverance we could potentially see a brighter world in which we can all live.

When I decided to make a significant change, this was dropping something which I thought was not benefiting me, I was met by my own fear projections of the future. I was sitting in my chiropractor's waiting room and deciding whether to leave the WhatsApp group all the people I had been involved with in life for the past 10+ years was a part of. Nothing personal against these guys all of whom I still am very fond of, but I couldn't see how my lifestyle and interaction with this group was at all benefiting me, agreed I had some bigger changes to make other than this, but this was still very significant. I surrendered to the feelings I was having to leave, dropped all fear projections right there and went for it. I left the group, and as you all may know, it's obvious on a WhatsApp group who's left. So, it was a big deal in my head to drop these fear projections. Within a matter of seconds, the song that came over on the radio in that waiting room was *Man in the Mirror*!

So, my trust in the process, the universe gave me a clear sign back immediately in life and real time (if there is such a thing). Amazing synchronicity and justification in my eyes.

And lo and behold, I think only one person from that group asked me, was I okay? Hahaha, I had never felt better.

My Why

It astounded me when I discovered my "why". It was stumbled upon on a morning drive to work. It came to me so clearly, my "why" was to me at least, why I was repetitively making the same mistakes. Why I was doing it helped me breakthrough to *Upgrade Me* mania and put in place some new why's, why I wanted to upgrade/change – improve my whole being.

My biggest issue for me was continual binge drinking and in turn, failing to secure the vows I promised to my wife. Now don't get me wrong, I love my wife dearly and would never intentionally hurt her, but I was! I couldn't see the damage because I justified my behaviour (drinking) above how she was made to feel. I would tell my wife and indeed myself, to give reason to this behaviour, 'you haven't lost your mum', or 'you haven't had a close family member pass away in your family, you don't know what it's like'. Another old favourite of mine would be, 'this is who I am', how pathetic an excuse I now think this was.

I gave myself a label – and believed it! And that is where many people's problems lie. Because they believe they can't change it. If you believe that label, then how can you change – this is you, right? WRONG! You are not a label, you are not your past, you are not your faults, bad habits or anything that justifies them (excuses). If you see these then change them at least. There were no excuses for me when I discovered my why. And I would like to take this opportunity to thank my wife, who I love so much and owe a lot to, for she never believed the label I gave myself, she never believed the excuses for letting her down. She believed in someone that was resonating deeply within me, waiting to come out. She stood by me for me to become my best.

My why was "unconditional love". This may sound or seem bizarre, but allow me to explain.

It became clear to me that my alcohol-drinking habits were formed a long time ago, way before my wife and I met. And because of my environment and seeing other people's relationship with alcohol, I accepted it as the norm; it was normal. Partly why I would say to my wife on occasions, 'This is who I am.' But it wasn't (this was a "like", I liked to drink). After my mother died the family dynamics changed for everyone. My father became a workaholic, doing his best to provide for the home and all his five children. Alcohol was a big part in taking the pain away of losing such an important person for my dad. The affect this had on me was not clear until I was 30 years old and realised that I lost that unconditional love my mum would have been able to bestow on me. I had affectively abandoned all ideas of unconditional love and replaced it with alcohol for acceptance within a group. I realised I couldn't see (the whole time) the true love my wife was trying to show to me because I was too well versed in being accepted with alcohol and the culture. I became someone that was not my true essence because I found a way to be accepted (without love) – drinking!

Hallelujah, I had an answer in my mind and it was a relief. I could do something about it. "Upgrade!"

Authenticity

Discovering who you are is key to upgrading. To become the real and genuine you can be daunting. You may know who that person is, or you may not. I had an inkling I was not the person I appeared to be to others because of the overwhelming feeling of discord in certain situations. My guise was not a true reflection of my internal voice, my intuition.

Upgrading yourself to show the true authentic you to the outside world will give your life balance, more happiness and more genuine love.

Imagine for a moment that you have been shut out from the outside world for the first five years of your life, and all you have ever known from the outside world was purely make-believe, imaginary and fictitious. When you would first see the world, it would seem bizarre and peculiar. The strangeness would make you feel uncomfortable and eldritch. As you would begin to observe the world and its ways, you would begin to breakdown the false views, beliefs and misconceptions that have entrenched themselves to your subconscious. You would need to adapt yourself. This is the same for you. If you have grown up listening to other people's opinions of you and copying other people to fit in, the veracity of your own behaviour, and indeed the makeup of your personality, will not be genuine. You cannot be the authentic you if you don't know who you are.

This can sound very daunting and perhaps a bit overwhelming in a sense of, "I must know who I am". But it needn't be. You don't need to go on a path of solitude and isolation to completely discover who you are. In fact, some recent research led by Alison Lenton, was written up in the *European Journal of Personality*, and would suggest the opposite when it comes to authenticity. Being social is good for you and can bring out some of your more authentic traits. Just be careful of the company you are keeping. As part of any upgrade, you want what's genuine to the label. You wouldn't want an Apple phone on the outside with backstreet parts on the inside. So being authentic for me would be aligning yourself with your actions, and reflecting your true intentions. Unalloyed in all situations, either social or in seclusion, would be the peak of authenticity of your character. You can upgrade purely by just discovering your own originality and being true to it. This is the authentic you.

It will become a pleasure to discover your own originality, along with your strengths, unlimited potential and making the possibility of an upgrade one step closer. You are original, one of a kind, your personality slightly tweaked just for you – now it's time to act authentically and accordingly to access your full potential and upgrade.

Be aware that there is a belief system based purely on "you" that exists within others. Depending on the level of time someone has spent with you, the experiences you have had together and the relationship between each other, there could be potentially as many "yous" as you have fingers and toes, in other people's minds.

This is likely to be because you have never found the true essence of your being, the authentic you! So, you have been many different people in the company of many individuals. Occasionally, when time elapses between the interactions of yourself and certain individuals, if you have significantly "changed", (become the more authentic you) it can be an odd experience. That certain individual has a belief system based on the past, which made up the old you, but since you have upgraded (grown) you cannot interact on that same level anymore (behave in the manner you previously did). The opinion of that individual should not be of any relevance to you just because they are basing you on the past. Simply move on and don't allow this to affect your "upgrade". It can be difficult if someone dislikes the new you, but with this upgrade, authenticity is what's key, and this should give you a high level of independence of knowledge about yourself. Don't allow anyone to define who you should be, not for any reason, especially based on the past. Even if you have knocked around with someone for 5–10 years, didn't see them for one reason or the next for a further 5–10 years but you kept in some intermittent contact, how much can they really claim to know you, or you know them?

Later in this book, I will give you my strategy to help guide you to achieve your upgrade. First off, I want you to build up the belief that an upgrade is truly possible. Therefore, I wanted to share with you some of my own personal issues. I am showing you a part of me, to give the perspective of an upgrade some substantiation. It is not some far-off dream or something out of the realms of possibility. Be unstoppable and gain positive momentum in your life, start with a bite-size-me list.

'It's always impossible until it's done' – Nelson Mandela

Nothing can hold you back from your originality but yourself; the mind is curious in its workings and will throw a lot of doubt and fear your way. The mind will make you question what you are doing! Ultimately, and without getting into the neuroscience of the brain, your mind has become comfortable, relaxed and does not want you to create new habits that are out of its comfort zones. However, you need to blast through these doubts if you want to achieve the upgraded version of yourself. Any upgrade (change) that you endeavour to succeed in must come from the authentic you, otherwise it is doomed to fail horribly and could backfire. Always use the power of the authentic you for positive returns, and do not use it to manipulate a person or situation for short-term gains. It won't last! So, make sure when you set out to achieve a certain goal, it's for the good of "you", it will benefit you in a positive way and will not have any detrimental effect to anybody else.

If part of your upgrade is to move out of any unhappy relationship, be it romantic, professional or friendships, and it will bring you more in accordance with the authentic you then it is for the best of both parties. It allows you to carry on with your upgrade and allows everyone to view your positive change. This will, in the long term, be positive for everyone involved.

Acceptance

The idea of an upgrade from one part of your being to another is hopefully a notion which resonates with you so well, that the explanations in this book jump out at you and sink deep into your consciousness. The gravitational pull into your new upgrade is gaining momentum and you are falling into a new and unknown cycle of events; you can almost sense a kind of rebirth is taking place with magical events being witnessed in front of your eyes. Accept this fully, embrace it without fear and allow things and events to take their course and begin to trust.

Embracing and accepting change is a must. An upgrade cannot take place if you hold onto things which no longer serve the person you are becoming.

Acceptance in the belief in yourself has grown, do not allow it to wilt and shrink away because of your own past or someone else's opinions of the new you. Embracing yourself fully, which entertains exactly who you have been previously as well as the person you are becoming. The positive does not exist alone, there is always a negative, accept this. How do I qualify this statement (in a positive sense), you can make a decision which your own heart feels is for the best (positive), yet there may very well be a negative outcome, or at least there is a fear of the negative outcome within your thought process, which prevents the positive decision taking place.

I'll take my own example; becoming my own boss, starting my own business. A definite positive move of the King on the chess board. This kind of set up and change in life circumstances cannot take place without accepting that failure is a possibility. Learning to accept that there are negative outcomes in decisions, and not trying to control everything down to the most finite of details is giving trust to the process and accepting fully the learning curve that will most certainly take place and, give you space to really begin to create without the fear of failure. The beauty of an outcome which you allowed to just be, is that you learn something new, about yourself, the process and the events which took place.

A conversation I had recently with someone to encourage them (as I believe in them myself) to start their own business made me think of this acceptance idea. They said this, 'I don't do failure, I am a perfectionist, so if I'm not ready I'm not going to do it'.

Without judging and just analysing this statement, would you not agree that this person has limited themselves purely because they cannot accept failure as part of the process?

When is the right time to do anything, at what point would you qualify to run your own business, or do anything for that matter? Acceptance runs deep into our lives and affects all aspects: personal, business, social interactions, hobbies, romance, financial, bereavements. The list is large. Accepting the positive as well as the negative and embracing it instead of it swallowing you up into a great big ball of fear, which affects you doing anything that is new, is a must.

Accept who you have been, accept who you are becoming and accept that for anything positive to take place, failure will always be by its side, ready to teach you for the best.

Accept this in print of an idea into your mind; you are great. Let it grow with all its outcomes and possibilities.

Sacrifice, discipline and potential:

For any new personal upgrade and growth to take place, there needs to be some improvements in honing and attaining skills which have not been so prevalent in your life. Everything in life is a skill learned, believe it or not, sacrifice is a skill that is learned. It can always seem that someone else has it all or it comes easy to them, but when you analyse their behaviour and routines, you will observe that sacrifice has played a significant part in their endeavours to succeed in what they are succeeding in. Now, if you analyse your own behaviour, does it have the same level of consistency in the endeavours you wish to win at?

Sacrifice: As part of your upgrade, practise honing the skill of sacrifice. When it is time to change/upgrade, when you feel your intuition tugging at you and swaying you in the direction of something new, this is the time you have to analyse what exactly needs to be done in order to go down this new path. So, sacrifice in itself will be what is carried out in order for you to make your way down the intuitive path of the unknown. Depending on which direction you will be going in for your upgrade, there is undoubtedly going to be something left behind, this is the sacrifice. Is it a behaviour, is it a character trait which no longer serves you? The illusion of this magnificent thing we call time, is always going to be part of the sacrifice stage of the upgrade, you will give up part of your "free" time to gain the space in your life for the upgrade me version of you. Time sacrifice is the development stage, if you don't sacrifice the time to hone the skill for the new upgraded version of yourself, how would you expect to succeed?

The sacrifice of many things may come into play overall, for the new you to arrive into your daily and present life. My personal sacrifice in order to make (a huge quantum leap) has been to give up alcohol. This has given me the time and space to hone my skills in the upgraded version of my new self. Without this sacrifice, I would most certainly be in the continual loop of the old me, wondering (yet not really wondering because I knew what needed to be done) how to advance to the stage of the new Upgrade Me! Sacrifice is a skill, why? Because it forces you to make decisions that change things. Making decisions is the precursor to the act of sacrifice, the skill being practised is making decisions. A by-product of the process of decision making is losing the fear factor that is at the forefront of your mind, just before a decision is made. By simply learning the skill of sacrifice (by actually practising it), you are practising and also honing the attributes/skills of decision-making and gaining confidence with learning you can make a decision, hence loosing fear of making decisions. Never be scared of making a decision and the outcome when your intuition is in play.

Discipline: This skill will be the backbone of your world and the new upgraded version of you. You have made the decision, sacrificed, and now it's time to be disciplined. Being able to be disciplined in the event of something, which will test your veracity of the new upgraded version of you is the ultimate test of discipline in your new character. The simple act of getting up and going to work is carried out by many millions of people around the world, but is it carried out with just routine? Done well, and with conscious thought, your alarm is set for the correct time to wake from your sleep, you have organised the night before all belongings required for the following days' work, clothes, lunch, keys, phone etc. This simple set of tasks is at its lowest form, discipline. But make no mistake, this done well sets up your day! These tasks carried out are the small areas of discipline in your daily life, which take just a little effort and preparation and give you the learning curve of discipline for the bigger parts of your life. It gives you a basis to work with and propel further onto bigger and larger life objectives; you need your discipline in all circumstances of life. From getting up and going to work to achieving large goals which require a lot more time and consistency of discipline. When you can discipline your mannerisms within your character to present yourself as your best version; this is a whole new skill. Learning to remain calm in a negative situation, learning to attune your reactions to better suit a positive outcome from a difficult day, takes discipline. Learning to sit and as previously mentioned, be content with your present moment and all it is within that moment, takes discipline. This is a skill, which needs to be practised from the minute small tasks of the day like setting your alarm and organising your belongings, to setting goals and sticking to the routines which require discipline and consistency to achieve them.

Potential: Your life is potential waiting to happen. You are bounded energy and are unsure of this energy's potential, like a spring under compression you are coiled up and raring to go, yet you are not springing forwards!

Once you recognise you are full of all this potential waiting to be released, focus on this. You need to become fully aware of your own life and its meaning for you. The potential you have as an individual is great, but only the purpose of belief can give you what is waiting to be released. Let your creative spirit come out once you hear the voice calling for change, to grow, to upgrade, sacrifice what is necessary and be disciplined to fulfil your full potential.

The Remarkable Mind

Never fear, your mind is near. Your mind is your greatest asset and the most priceless resource you have in your life. If you have nothing else but the workings of your mind, you need no more.

Your mind is your factory, your processing plant – the machine behind your body. There's a saying, you are what you eat. And this is true, however – I would prefer to say you are what you feed your mind. Information leads to transformation. Inform yourself with good quality knowledge – knowledge about food perhaps, or fitness/health, practise that information and it will lead to transformation. Why be unhealthy and overweight, which will cause you health problems, when you can be healthy?

Anything you do is your responsibility – so start being consciously responsible for what you choose to watch, what you choose to read, and what you choose to believe in.

Belief systems stem from social constructs which lead people into different ways of thinking, therefore their beliefs. From a social housing estate to central London apartments, they will have a definite belief system that is miles apart! This is personal belief system, and habitual belief system.

This is not to say the belief systems of "someone" from a council estate (I am from a council estate) is any less important than those of more affluent areas, but make no mistake, the difference it can make is huge. The impact on life expectancy is probably the best, and most clear example I can give for the differentiation of the two. The belief system of someone from a more affluent construct of life to that of someone in less fortunate circumstances has an actual impact on their length of life, and it's not all down to money! It's how you see yourself, your belief in your own self that's key. It's time to "upgrade" once you recognise your own potential and self-worth.

The fundamental belief systems of the main (the collective, the whole) would be different from one set of constructs to the next. Of course, there are always anomalies (be the anomaly). The environment which the individual lives can dictate someone's thinking, therefore their belief system, therefore their limitations of themselves. The continual loop of successive generations doing the same thing because of how they are taught and what they are taught and how they see themselves. The cycle can only be broken if someone decides to think and believe differently, otherwise society stays the same, moreover, you stay the same. The person who breaks this cycle will teach their children or others this knowledge, and as long as it's applied, change in the collective can begin with the new generation, so on and so forth.

No matter when, at some point in your life you will need to break away from blame, take responsibility and move forward (where you have come from). And your mind is the place it will start! You can learn anything, do anything – be anything

Learn this – plasticity, the adaptability of an organism to changes in its environment or differences between its various habits. Your remarkable mind can adapt and change to many different scenarios, environments and settings, all due to the brain's plasticity. Its ability to change – upgrade. This is the tool you will learn to use to give the change in your life that you so desire.

Ownership

Your beautiful life on this planet is yours and no one else's. Yes, we must give thanks to our parents for their coming together and helping to bring us here – but they themselves do not own or control you. You alone, take forth the direction you wish to go in. The power you have is all in your decisions today that will give you an outcome that is more gratifying and fulfilling tomorrow. Love your life and love yourself – I cannot stress this enough.

Every waking hour you have, you can consciously create – so create beautifulness and own it. It's yours, be proud of it. Small steps in the right direction are still steps in the right direction. Never falter away from discipline upon yourself – only you can choose wisely, or badly. So, when a wise decision requires you to be disciplined, be disciplined.

You own all your decisions, some I agree will not be as profound as others, but nonetheless, whatever it is, it is yours! A bad mood does not justify a bad decision or angry response, that's just an excuse and a lack of discipline.

People of this world – I want to give you a gift. A gift of belief. Just imagine for one second that this book you hold is that belief. And no matter where you go you will have it. Believe in yourself. Believe in a better you and a better tomorrow.

Be, life.

Belief.

You are life, so believe in yourself.

Learn principles of character first: What are your principles?

Patience: Having this as a "principle" character trait requires practice; it's not a given that you will be born with the virtue of patience. Learning / practicing this skill set and acquiring it as a "principle of character" will generate a whole host of subsidiary skills, which will be highlighted as it comes to the fore to benefit you as a whole. Patience in general will give you the opportunity to also practise being calm. Being calm will help you to keep / remain focused. So, from one principle of character, "oh he's such a patient man", you can develop your character to be a lot stronger in testing situations. Always remind yourself of the upgrade you so wish to create, it won't happen by accident. "Principles of your character" can help you to develop the necessary skill sets; to help you obtain the Upgrade Me version of yourself. What principles do you want your character to be moulded by?

BELIEF
Upgrade Me requires you to believe in yourself to such a level that the life and upgrade you are looking to achieve, must be unwavering under all circumstances. This is ultimately only generated if you have reached the level of authenticity. If you can't be authentic or haven't reached this level yet, when testing times come, it may rock your foundations and you can lose faith in your vision. But don't despair, if your true desire is to "upgrade" (change) then when the testing times come, if you feel like you are rocked into submission and all is lost, you begin to think this is unattainable! Revert to this!

G: gaining

R: recognisable

O: observable

W: Wisdom

Grow through your storms and take from it something useful, add it to your armoury in preparation for the next storm. Nothing in life will sail perfectly all the time, you can have years of so-called plain sailing, but if you have no belief in who you are (your authenticity), when testing times come around it will be hard to get through. But if you have unwavering belief in yourself and your "upgrade", the storms will pass, and you will "grow". You will be able to take something tangible from that situation, and go wisely into the next phase of life.

POETIC STRATEGY AND THE LOOP YOU WANT TO BE IN:

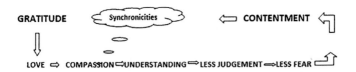

This is a beautiful loop and works beautifully once understood. However, I am open-minded (open to all possibilities) to the fact someone could look at this and say, 'No that's not right!' And they may want to say there is 'x' in between compassion and understanding, or 'x' in between less fear and contentment. But through my own application of the cycle, I have less judgement of the opinions of others and I can be open-minded to the contribution (open to all possibilities) someone can make to improve this loop. Just like adding new circuitry to the brain and signalling a new gene to work in our bodies, all contributions are welcome as long as they benefit the loop for the positive balance of nature.

1. Gratitude: This, for me, has been compelling, being thankful at the end of each day and as soon as I wake from my night's sleep (which isn't currently much, living with a four-year-old and a one-year-old) has transformed almost everything in my life. If you can learn this skill as I did, hone it until it becomes a natural part of your day, you begin to see your whole day in a new light. So, what does this all mean if you're reading and trying to understand this for the first time? From my own perspective, giving thanks in the morning first that you have awoken for a new day, you have the opportunity to lead the day if you just give thanks, and consciously be aware of your thought processes. It can sound like I am an annoyingly happy person who lives in cloud cuckoo land. But this is not the case. I still get annoyed, upset and occasionally angry. But my deployment of gratitude is my first port of call as I wake, it's my choice to actively choose to think in a thankful and grateful manner. I give thanks that I have awoken, I give thanks that I have been in my bed all night safely (blessings of a home), I give thanks for the beautiful family I have. Simple things which were always in my face, but which I never always consciously recognised as being abundantly wonderful things in my life. This then sets the tone for my day. I feel the love for the things which are important to me and are most precious. From this simple skill, I transport all those positive feelings through the entire day; I am grateful for the smallest things which become beautifully, a part of my day. The trees I see on my journey, the weather I am experiencing at that particular time (I genuinely love the rain), the birds which appear to be random, but I recognise as not so random in my day. My gratitude spreads to everything within my day that I consciously choose to activate it upon. This way, there is a lot less space for negativity to create a space in my mind and take over my day. As my day draws to a close, I give thanks for all the things I endured through my day, I reflect on my moments I was not so conscious of and I am grateful for the day. I look forward to the next day with enthusiasm to create a whole new experience I would again, be grateful for. Learn the gratitude skill, as everything in life is a skill learned; do not limit yourself and think this is not "you", it's a skill that requires attention. Activate it, learn it, use it! Now, what can you start feeling grateful for in your life, picture it in your mind and feel it. Practise this daily, don't worry where you "think" you are starting from on this, just start! It will grow!

2. Love: From gratitude, we are led to love. Love is said to be the greatest power in the universe and on planet earth. The feeling of true love, a feeling that will shine from within, begins to expand and grow as you learn the true essence of yourself. You become so overwhelmed with this emotion it melts away the rocky core you once had, and you begin to feel liberated. Loving yourself and your authenticity will make you shine even brighter. You will begin to affect those around you and whom you come into contact with as your demeanour will be love. Love spreads like wildfire once you recognise it. You will hold yourself accountable for your actions even on the smallest of things, and if it doesn't resonate with love, you will not be doing things against yourself or anybody else. Love will make you see things in a new light and from a different perspective; you can no longer look away from things that don't sit right with you. You will step into a new power called love and it will transcend you from the shadowy being you once was. It will give you peace within yourself and towards others. Love will become the cloak that embodies you, plants its seed and sprouts from within; everybody will see it and you most certainly will feel the change that love will bring to your transcendence.

3. Compassion: Your newfound transcendence of love into your being will have a new close friend along with it, compassion. For once in your life, when you get something and it comes with a "catch", you will have compassion as a new string to your bow, not a hard-to-swallow bitter pill. You will be sensitive to things of a delicate nature, and deal with situations which offer you a chance to turn away, but you tackle it with a compassionate heart. Difficult situations and difficult people are best viewed compassionately.

4. Understanding: Being able to understand someone, or a situation, is a vital life skill you should prominently and actively pursue to master. Mastery in anything is only attained through continual practice, perseverance and attention to detail. Be aware when people are talking to you and listen well, really make them feel they are understood. Acquiring this skill lets you understand for yourself that other people have needs, feeling what they feel can be a side kick to this "understanding" skill and allow you to see things from their perspective. This will enlighten you to a whole new world (once again and not for the first time on this journey) and make you a better, more rounded person.

5. Less Judgement: Understanding someone and their needs and being able to see things from their perspective with a loving and compassionate heart, will allow you to make less judgements on people, their lifestyles, their backgrounds and their circumstances. Your heart and mind will be open once you are understanding, and you will have less reason to judge! This will allow you to be more and more accepting in your life, if you can accept people and judge less it can ultimately only make you a happier person. Less complaining, less gossip and less stressful thoughts.

6. Less fear: Fear of the unknown is probably one of the biggest propagators in people's lives that cause them not to change. Once you have gone through the above format as I have in my own life, you will begin to notice you can make better decisions in life based on a very grounded, solid reasoning process, which does not yield due to fear projections of the mind coming into play. Your new decisions in life will be based all upon the authenticity of your newfound self (your true essence) and will reflect a more balanced view in your life.

7. Contentment: For me at least, I have endured many battles of being content. I have always looked externally to fill the joy in my life, whether it be alcohol, going out to socialise or even comfort eating. But once I came to a point of less fear, I could make decisions that were actively better for myself, without the fear of being judged if I didn't go to that party or go to that family event. Not everything needs my attention if it doesn't serve me, and I am happy in the decision due to less fear. This gave space for me to recognise the things I am content about. Looking to gain some popularity down the pub, or always being involved in a night out no longer served me and my "upgrade". Gratitude for the pleasures I've always had but never held dear enough to feel content, was staring me in the face. Contentment is balance in my life and serving my family, and all their needs. I now actively pursue my healthy hobbies, serve my family and their needs, and keep my mind happy with new knowledge.

8: Amazing Synchronicities: Once you have developed a freedom in your mind based on the attributes and skills from the above loop, you will begin to see that things in your life start working for you. The power of the universe begins to show you signs you're on the right path; it will support you in your endeavours and it will help you trust more in your own intuition and internal voice of good. This is the prize of the loop system above (as far as I can tell) to reward you with something supportive for the path you are now on. These amazing synchronicities can be boldly obvious or sometimes just a little more subtle. The more subtle ones will tend to find your awareness only when you look back on things with hindsight. The bold and obvious can leave you astounded and in amazement with what the power of the universe can do and show you. The loop begins again from here as you are in pure gratitude for this support you have been offered with no obvious efforts of your own. It's only when you reflect on the "feelings" you have be having (hence the above cycle/loop I have come to recognise) you realise how powerful your emotions can be, especially when they are in a state of positivity, i.e. gratitude. Whilst writing this book, I saw a truck parked as I was stuck in traffic approaching a roundabout, it said on the side of it, "paradigm", which immediately made me think *paradigm shift*. Exactly what I have done to change my life and "upgrade me", is a paradigm shift. At this point I gave thanks to the universe for sending me such a nice message, allowing me to feel grateful and ultimately content I am on the right path. At this point of thanking the universe the traffic began to move, and as I approached nearer the roundabout, a truck came from the right on the roundabout and pulled off at the junction I was sitting at waiting to get on. Above the main windscreen of the truck it said, "TE ALL", which I read as "Tell All". The sign from the universe made me laugh in amazement and in awe of the beautifully constructed message. Paradigm shift, tell all. Tell all to shift their paradigm, and create a new and better you;

keep writing the book and keep expressing it in the way you are, to convey to the reader a way of changing their lives.

Apart from reading this book multiple times to gain the essence of its meaning, here are my strategy tips to help you succeed in achieving your upgrade:

- Follow the meaning of this book, and similar books to stay focused and give perspective
- Highlight key areas in this book that resonate with you and make them stand out
- Create a bite-size-me list, without fail, and breakdown who you are currently
- Create a list of words/characteristics you would want your new upgrade to reflect – work on one point at a time and master it – it's for the good of you
- Keep a track record of progress – list of achievements to help you feel positive when times are tough
- Keep this book with you
- Memorise the chapter headings – poetic strategy – keeps you focused and gives something to come back and pay attention to, if your mind is deterring you from your goal. Something easily repeated in your mind can help bring you back to the essence – and give you that kick of BELIEF
- Learn this short poem, considering it has chapter headings in there. Each chapter heading will have uniqueness to you – things you've highlighted in that chapter – so learning this poem will help remind you of what it is that resonates with you.

We gather ourselves from our "remarkable mind", to understand what's deep inside.

How can it be this "bitesize me" has fallen from the sky and come to be?

In what way has "my why" formed? So, I asked myself, "what right do I have to be miserable?"

The "ownership" I give is mine, and mine alone, to create a life just like "time for another phone"

It is that quick, so "it's on you",
"Coming away from yourself" is what you must do
To create a new, how great will this be, touching the flower like a dependable bee,
As strong as ox and as authentic as a tree.
The wind will blow but you shall not wither, as flexible as the smallest branch and as strong as the widest trunk
Your branches will grow, and your roots will spread firm, how great will this be to finally see, your true form

Your authenticity
U: upload
P: personal
G: gratitude daily
R: rehearse
A: attributes that
D: define the visons
E: equal to your authenticity
M: measurable and meaningful
E: equilibrium and balance

The Art of self-discovery
This is ultimately what upgrade me is all about, discovering who you truly are. It is, your own art. The beauty of this is that it is akin to a rabbit in a magician's hat, there appears to be nothing and then suddenly, a rabbit is magically pulled out. When you look deep inside yourself, from what once there appeared to be nothing, now out from the darkness there is something anew. You begin to discover there is more to your being and your understanding of life, and its wonders magnify! You will see things differently. The art of self-discovery is completely yours, unique to you and your life, your perceptions and perspectives. Learning to listen to your inner guide/voice is the key to grasping the paintbrushes of your soul, and painting the art of your life onto the canvas of the world. The "you" you have lived with your whole life, if this is a misprint of society's design upon you then it's time to delve deep inside that rabbit whole and pull out your gift

and present it to the world. You are the artist of your own life, and you create the art within the discovery of your true authentic self. "The art of self-discovery", it's yours! Just follow the signposts of life to guide you, the small internal messages you feel, and the rest is all yours. You will find gifts that are more tangible and real than you could ever have imagined possible, a belief within will become unshakable and you will "grow". Upgrade me is the new you!

There is no perfection to be attained from this, in fact it's more of a realisation. Although dissecting yourself to get to the core of your authenticity is difficult, through peeling back your layers of "likes", and discarding what is not necessary as to accompany you on the upgrade, it is far more beneficial to just realise that these things were a part of you and in a funny kind of way, has contributed to your journey of self-discovery. This is part of the process in order to upgrade. Never neglect what you were in such a way, that you can't recognise the process it has played in your life. The ying and yang is an interconnected circle, the relationship of opposite and contrary forces are complementary to each other. You can give rise to a new you, but only through the old you; it had its purpose and now it's time to go further in your development as a person and a human being. Be accepting in your own art of self-discovery and accept your past, its flaws and its connection to you.

Thanking you:

If you have reached this far in the book, well done. This may be your first book you have ever read, or it could just be the start of a process which allows you to actively pursue other like-minded books which support your endeavours to be a better you. To Upgrade. Whatever it may be, I thank you sincerely for reading this book and entertaining its ideas. Truthfully, I believe from writing this book I have managed to upgrade further in my own process, deepen my own connection to this world, but most importantly, deepen my own spirit which lies within. I trust myself to make the right decision, which includes putting other people's feelings before mine. My passion to improve has led me on a wonderful journey; how to convey this all in one single book would be masterful, as it would be endless. The passion to improve has inspired me to write, something I felt for a long time but never ever got the enthusiasm enough to even begin. But once I felt the need to write, it was a case of "I must get these thoughts and feelings out to the world". I hope you have sincerely enjoyed this booked and it manages to inspire you to envisage a better you, and kick-starts you into a new life. The world truly is your oyster, and it has a lot to teach you about you! Discovering who you are deep within, and allowing that authenticity to grow and shine will be the greatest gift you will ever discover and use.

Thank you to my wife who has, by and large, been my earth angel. Someone who has stood by me through thick and thin, and given me the strength and courage to be able to make the changes I have in my life.

Thanks to my dad who once gave me a list of words as a child, a list that was almost like a guide to attain good character; "learn how to learn", and "persevere" were just two on that list. I remember it very well, yet in the early adult part of my life that went amiss, but perhaps the word "persevere" is exactly what I have done in all that I have ever done, they were wise words that I still use today. Thank you, dad.

Closing Statements

Just like a lawyer convincing the jury of a case in the final stages, I would like to leave you with this.

If you know you have one chance in life to do something great, could you truly let it slip out of your grasp? Have you grasped how great you can be yet?

You are a magnificent being with the potential to be greater than you currently are. Don't accord greatness to material wealth only; being a great parent or being a great employee is what is tangible in this world. Materialism comes and materialism goes, it's lovely when you have something nice and you have worked hard for it but did you do it with great character, did you do it with pride and passion, without misplaced hate along the way for someone else? Upgrade yourself to a level beyond what is material, and make yourself grow as a person. Put yourself in a testing situation to reveal your greatness and your character, give yourself time to be great. Take on new challenges and test your mind's capacity to learn new things, new skills, meet new people and create new experiences instead of the familiar day-to-day routine. Keep things fresh and upgrade. Continually refresh the pages of your mind like the open tabs on your computer.

Allow yourself some time to grow from the current situations and environment you are currently in, because it takes time to make long-lasting changes which benefit you. The sincerity of the changes that are being made will be felt deep inside and make the feeling of contentment flourish; this will give you strength to continue on your path, to upgrade in the face of criticism and backlash. Although change is a must, most people fear change as it presents new challenges which removes them completely out of their comfort zone. Even if it is you who is doing the changes in your life in order to upgrade it, it will present new ways for the familiar people in your life to interact with you. This can cause the backlash, as it is inadvertently forcing them out of their own comfort zones. Don't allow this to affect your upgrade and do it anyway!

Make the life you wish for possible, and upgrade today. *Upgrade Me* is here to teach you that life must be tackled with a creative mind and an open heart. Combine the two and you will naturally start to learn all about what power you possess.

Go with love for yourself.